Lymphedema Diet

A Smart and Sustainable Plan Centered on Inflammation and Weight Control

Thaddeus Conklin

By reading this notice, the reader agrees that
under no circumstances is the author responsible
for any losses, direct or indirect, that are
incurred as a result of the use of information
contained within this book, including, but not
limited to, errors, omissions, or inaccuracies.

Table of Contents

Introduction

Right now you might be dealing with lymphedema and for that let me share my condolences. I can't change whatever may have happened in the past that ultimately brought you to this book, but hopefully, I can help brighten your future a little bit. At the time of writing, there is no cure for lymphedema, but there are things you can do to help improve the condition.

That's what the aim is going to be for this book. I want to focus on the things we can control to help improve whatever the situation is that you currently find yourself in. The area that we're going to hone in on is going to be your nutrition.

No matter who you are or what condition you have, nutrition is a powerful thing. It has the power to change the cells in your body for better or for worse. This is why the phrase you are what you eat has always stood out to me.

The foods that you're eating today will help to create new cells that will literally comprise who you are. That is crazy to stop and think about. So this isn't something that only people with a certain condition should care about, everyone should care about the topic of nutrition.

Sadly very few do for one reason or another, and it has caused a wide variety of health problems throughout our society. You're different though, and I know that because you're taking the time to read this book.

This shows me that you care enough to want to make changes in your life. You just might need some guidance and direction for how you should approach things and I'm happy to assist with that.

Chapter 1: What is Lymphedema?

Lymphedema is the swelling of the arms, legs, neck, and face due to the body being unable to properly move fluid throughout the system. This occurs due to lymph nodes that have been damaged or removed thus not allowing the lymphatic system to properly do its job. Lymphedema can occur for multiple reasons.

One of these is a cancer patient who has some of the lymph nodes removed as part of their treatment. Injury, infection, and genetic mutations are other causes that can lead to lymphedema. Common symptoms of lymphedema are heaviness or a full feeling in the affected areas such as the extremities.

You may also notice that your clothes fit tighter than they usually do. And as I mentioned in the introduction, there is no cure for lymphedema as of the writing of this book. However, there are various treatments you can do to help manage your symptoms. These things include exercise, diet, compression wraps, and massages.

No Matter What Got You Here, You're Striving to Move Forward

One of the difficult things about lymphedema is that it can occur through no fault of your own. Think of the main causes of lymphedema that I listed: cancer treatment, injury, injection, and genetic mutations. Sure some lifestyle choices over some time could lead to cancer, such as smoking leading to lung cancer.

A lot of people though get diagnosed with cancer and there's seemingly no explanation of anything to pin it on. You don't have any control over your genetics either, so that leaves injury and infection. Most people are not intentionally trying to go out and get injured or have an infection occur.

So it may very well be the case that you're dealing with something that unfortunately happened to you through an accident or through no fault of your own. That can be a tough thing to deal with. No matter what has brought you to this point in time, you can not change the past.

I know it's painful and I'm sure the thought of, "Why me?", has crossed your mind many times. I'm truly sorry that this is something you're dealing with. What I can tell you is something that's helped me through difficult times is to focus on changing my future through the actions that I'm taking today and to let go of the past.

It's not easy to do this, but it's a strong way that you can make progress. It's hard to move forward when we're still trying to process what we're dealing with in the present. However, I know that you are wanting to make progress in your future.

So whenever things get tough, think about the future that you want to create for yourself. Think about how you want to be able to move freely, willingly, and intentionally. Picture being able to put on your clothes every day without a struggle.

When times are tough and even though it's tough to do, I want you to focus on that. Thinking in this manner will give you the best chance of seeing success. You won't just automatically write things off because you don't think they'll work for you.

Instead, you'll stay more optimistic and hopeful and give it a shot. If you at least try, then you give yourself a chance to change. No matter what past diet failures you've had previously, I want you to leave those behind so you can focus on the

better future you can create for yourself by
following through on this plan.

Chapter 2: Best Nutrition Practices for Lymphedema

Similar to how there's no cure for lymphedema, there's no one best approach for nutrition when it comes to lymphedema. You may think this is a bad thing. Wouldn't you want a set way of eating to ensure you get the best results possible for this condition?

In theory, yes that would be the ideal scenario, but that isn't the case. It's not all bad though, pretend there was a best practice for how to eat with lymphedema. Let's say this approach involved food or practices that you hated and you could barely stand the thought of this diet plan anymore to the point where you'd rather deal with your symptoms in other ways.

Since there is no best approach, there's more flexibility in how you can approach your nutrition so that way you enjoy it. This way you'll be able to do it for the rest of your life without thinking twice about it and before you know it, it will be a fully ingrained habit. Even though there's not one specific best way to go about things, there are a couple of things we want to make sure we're doing, which I'll talk about right now.

The Two Main Things You Need to Focus On

When it comes to your diet, research shows that although there may not be a best approach for lymphedema, there are some things you can do to improve the situation. The first is to improve your BMI. There is research to indicate that as BMI increases, the symptoms of lymphedema will worsen.

Thus by lowering your BMI, you can help to lessen your symptoms. BMI stands for body mass index and it is very simple in terms of what it is. It's a ratio of your weight to your height. Based on what that ratio is, you'll get a number. That number will place you in one of five different categories:

- Underweight
- Healthy/Normal
- Overweight
- Obese
- Severely Obese

A BMI that is higher than 40 is considered to be severely obese. A BMI of 30-40 would put an individual in the obese category, and 25-30 puts someone in the overweight range. As an example, let's say someone is 6 feet tall and weighs 250 pounds.
This person's BMI would come out to about 34. You can calculate your BMI by plugging your height and weight into an online calculator. So if this person has lymphedema, has a BMI of 34, and they are able to improve their BMI to 28, their lymphedema symptoms should improve.

The way that you can improve your BMI is by losing weight. Therefore, losing weight by a healthy means is going to be an important part of improving your symptoms. Don't get me wrong, BMI is not the end all be all because it doesn't take muscle mass into consideration.

Muscle mass weighs more than fat and there are plenty of athletes that would be considered overweight by BMI standards. For the general population and for someone who is looking to improve lymphedema symptoms, this will be a good indicator to see if you're trending in the right direction. This is why one of the first things you should do is measure your BMI so that you know what your starting point is. It will be hard to correlate your symptoms improving if you don't even know what your original starting point was.

Eating Foods that Reduce Inflammation

The other thing that research does show is that eating foods that help to reduce inflammation can be beneficial for people with lymphedema. One of the main food types that help to reduce inflammation is going to be foods rich in Omega-3 fatty acids. Omega 3 fatty acids are anti-inflammatory to the body and are commonly found in foods such as nuts and fish.

On the other hand, you have Omega 6 fatty acids. A lot of Omega-6 fatty acids are found in foods that people tend to eat a lot of such as chips, candy bars, and other sweets and fast food items. Omega-6s are inflammatory to the body and putting an unnecessary amount of extra stress on the body is not something that needs to happen when you compile that with lymphedema.

Therefore, by focusing on eating less inflammatory foods and more anti-inflammatory foods, you could improve your symptoms. Here is a list of foods that we'll want to incorporate into the plan if possible:

- Salmon
- Tuna
- Mackerel
- Walnuts
- Pecans
- Lentils
- Blueberries
- Raspberries
- Blackberries
- Leafy Green Vegetables
- Coconut and Olive Oil
- Flax and Chia Seeds

This isn't a comprehensive list, but I want it to open your mind to help set the tone for what this diet plan should at least partially be composed of. A pattern that you'll notice is that these foods are wholesome, meaning that they don't contain ingredients. They are what they are.

For example, blueberries are just blueberries, there's nothing else to them. There are no preservatives, food dyes, or anything of that nature that you'll typically find in simple carbohydrate foods. Many simple carbohydrate foods you'll find will contain a long list of ingredients to help make the food last longer and make it taste better.

Take for instance a breakfast pastry, the taste is addicting so we'll continue to come back for more, and it's loaded with simple sugars and preservatives neither of which are going to be helpful for lymphedema. However, it will ensure that the food can last for a long time before it goes bad. This makes things easier for companies to sell because they don't have such a short time frame from which they can sell that food item.

Therefore, we want to focus on eating less of the simple sugars and high fatty food items, and more wholesome foods. A good general rule of thumb that you can employ is to look at the ingredient list. You may not know if a specific food is anti-inflammatory or not.

However, if you see a long ingredient list, chances are good that the food is not going to be helpful for your lymphedema. If the food item doesn't contain additional ingredients such as brown rice or quinoa, then chances are good that the food item will help to fight against inflammation. This isn't always going to be the case, for example, almonds contain Omega-6 fatty acids, but almonds are going to provide a lot more nutritional value for you compared to the fat you'll get from a slice of cheese pizza.

Another example is other foods that contain a small ingredient list, but are still derived from natural sources such as oat milk. So look for food items that have short ingredient lists as a general rule. This is why this simple rule is effective. You need to be able to follow something that's easy and not confusing.

If you're out and about, you need a rule you can follow to know if you should eat certain foods and avoid others. Your default needs to be resorting to the ingredient list. So if you're at a party and there's a food platter that contains chips, cookies, crackers, grapes, carrots, broccoli, and bell peppers, then you should avoid the chips, cookies, and crackers.

You should instead be snacking on the grapes, carrots, broccoli, and bell peppers. The chips, cookies, and crackers will increase inflammation and work against the symptoms you're already feeling with lymphedema. Meanwhile, the other foods will act as anti-inflammatories and help with your lymphedema symptoms.

The Overall Game Plan

With these two components in mind, we need to focus on improving our BMI and doing so by means of eating anti-inflammatory foods whenever possible. This will create the most ideal scenario for improving symptoms via diet. However, doing what should be done isn't necessarily the best thing to do in all situations.

For example, it might be ideal to eat foods that reduce inflammation as much as possible, but what if you're not able to sustain that? What if you really enjoy grabbing lunch with your friends or having a burger and chips on a cookout? It can kind of make it seem like you're either choosing between lymphedema or being miserable with what you eat.

This is why we must infuse one more aspect into this plan which is going to be sustainable factors. What I mean by this is eating foods that you enjoy so that way you can continue with this plan for a long time to come. Seriously, what does it matter if you know you should eat anti-inflammatory foods, but you don't do it because you eat them all of the time so you grow to loathe them?

People need variety in their lives. When we do the same thing day in and day out at work, what happens? We get bored! We want to do something else even if that new task isn't particularly thrilling.

Changing the pace can have a big impact on productivity at work, and the same principle applies to your diet. It will help to keep things feeling fresh and you'll be able to reward yourself with something you'll look forward to for the effort that you've been putting in. Typically when it comes to foods that people enjoy, they tend to not be that healthy.

Eating foods that are unhealthy may seem counterproductive to what we're trying to accomplish. It may seem that you will have a hard time improving your BMI if you're eating junk food. This is a common misconception and it's something that holds a lot of people back from making the progress that they want to see. Let's break down how it is that you actually go about improving your BMI.

How to Improve Your BMI

As I mentioned earlier, to improve your BMI all you have to do is lose weight. This is guaranteed to work up to a certain point since BMI is simply a height-to-weight ratio. You can't change your height, but you can lower your weight thereby improving your BMI.

I say up to a certain point because if you lose too much weight, now you're considered to be underweight and that isn't ideal either. So the real question becomes, how does someone lose weight? Most people would say you lose weight by eating healthy or by eating clean.

That answer comes from a good place, but it is not true. There have been people who have literally eaten primarily junk food to prove that losing weight is not about eating healthy, it's about something else. That something else is consuming less energy than you're burning off.

The energy that you're burning off in a given day is known as your metabolism. You need to eat fewer calories than what your metabolism is burning off to put your body in an energy deficit. This means you're providing your body with less energy than it needs to sustain itself.

This is where your body will then get the extra energy it needs to make up for the deficit from your fat stores, and this is how you lose weight. Conversely, your body only needs so much energy, so what happens when you provide your body with more energy (aka calories) than your body needs? It will store those extra calories as fat for a day later on when food is scarce and extra energy is needed.

More than likely you have access to food so it isn't scarce, but your body doesn't know that. It only knows how much food you're eating. Your body has to prepare for times when food might not be as available, and that's the benefit of fat storage.

It's what allowed people to survive back in the hunter-and-gather days. Like it or not, this is how our bodies work to gain and lose weight. Notice I didn't say anything about eating a certain type of food or avoiding a different type of food.

That's because in order to lose weight, there's nothing that's required for you to eat to lose weight. Conversely, there's nothing you have to completely give up in order to lose weight. So why then is society in general so obsessed with clean eating to lose weight?

Well for starters, the idea isn't bad in theory. Clean foods are more nutrient-dense. This means that you're going to get more calories on less volume of food.

Simple sugars, high-fat foods, or foods that contain empty calories typically contain a high amount of calories but the portion size of the food is small. For example, a slice of pizza might be 450 calories. That's not a lot of food for 450 calories.

Meanwhile, you'd have to eat a lot of vegetables, chicken, rice, or fruit for example to reach that same 450 calories. You're going to get a lot more full off of 450 calories worth of rice than you would from 450 calories of pizza. This is where eating healthy foods will benefit you.

You're going to have to eat less calories than you typically do in order to start losing weight. By filling up the majority of your diet with healthy foods, you'll be able to make the most of the calories that you do have. If you comprise the majority of your calories with junk food like pizza, they will go very quickly.

However, it's a mistake to think that your diet should consist only of healthy foods because that can only last for so long. Eventually, you'll get sick of it and quit on your plan. This is the exact reason why most diets don't work.

People go from eating fast food and dessert on a regular basis to suddenly stopping cold turkey. Those are some hard habits to break if you've been eating that way for years and years, which is why I'm preaching balance here. Knowing that you need to strike a balance is one thing, but what kind of a ratio should you strive for between healthy foods and not-so-healthy foods?

90/10 Rule

When it comes to sticking a balance with the types of foods you're eating, a good balance that I've found is to stick with following the rules 90% of the time and then being a little more loose the remaining 10% of the time. In this case, that means sticking with anti-inflammatory foods and other clean foods 90% of the time and the remaining 10% you can fill in however you please. This is great because it gives you wiggle room for when social events inevitably pop up.

It gives you a chance to keep things loose on the weekends when you likely want to relax. What

I've tended to notice is that it's easier to stick with a plan during the week when you're in the routine of going to work. When the weekends hit, things can be more challenging because you're out of your routine.

The day is more open and less focused. There are more social events that go on. This is when you'll be more likely to enjoy yourself a bit.

Now imagine if you didn't build in this 10%. You'd be resisting temptation consistently and that's hard to do. Then when you crack, you'll feel guilty for what you ate.

Instead, the 90/10 rule allows you to eat delicious foods guilt-free because it's a necessary part of the game plan to lower your BMI. The thing about this rule is that it's flexible. 90/10 might not be the perfect fit for you.

You might do better with an 85/15 or 80/20 split. The thing you have to understand is that you don't have to be perfect. It can be hard to change that way of thinking because that's likely how you've been ingrained to approach your health and fitness.

If you're not able to give 100%, then it's not worth doing. That is definitely false. Even if you follow a rule of 80% staying on top of things and 20% whatever you want, that's still an improvement and that's what matters.

The other consideration for this rule is that you can build your way up. If your ideal ratio is 90/10 for example, you might only be eating healthy 50% of the time right now. It's not a good idea to jump directly from 50% straight to 90%. Instead, you can work on gradually building your way up.

You could start by going up to a 60/40 split for the first week. Then the following week, you could take things up another notch and go 70/30. You could continue to improve things until you get to 90/10.

In practical terms what does this look like? How can you know if you're eating the right ratio or if you're indulging a bit too much? Well, let's use a hypothetical example with an individual who needs to eat 1,850 calories per day in order to lose weight.

This means that roughly 1,665 of those 1,850 calories on any given day need to come from clean sources. That's not a whole lot on any given day, which is why it makes sense to save those calories throughout the week. Let them add up into something that will give you more flexibility for when you need it the most.

After 5 days, this would accumulate to 925 calories, which is a good amount. You'd have enough calories at that point to eat a meal containing whatever you wanted. Or you could wait 6 days and accumulate 1,110 calories.

Maybe keeping up with calories isn't your thing. You instead can approach things in a slightly different yet still effective way. You could have 90% of the meals you eat be on point and the remaining 10% be from whatever you want.

If you average 3 meals per day, this means over one week, you're consuming 21 meals. This means that roughly 19 of your 21 meals need to be healthy meals with an emphasis on inflammation-reducing foods to help with lymphedema symptoms. Again remember though, this is going to be the most ideal way to go about things, but work your way up to this point.

Right now, let's say someone is currently only eating the way they ideally should be 50% of the time. This means that about 10-11 of their meals are not what they should be and the other 10-11 are. This is a starting point though.

This person could work on improving from 10-11 up to 12-13 and so on and so forth. This person would gradually work to improve things steadily week-by-week until they reach a point that they are satisfied with and feel like they can maintain. For some people, 90% might be too much and they might feel more comfortable with 80%.

Remember, making progress is better than trying to be spot-on all of the time. So if you improve from wherever you're starting from, that is something to celebrate. This can be a big mental hurdle for people to get over.

You think of where you should ideally be and if your choices don't align with that, we can beat ourselves up over it. I want you to think about how long you've been eating a certain way. For some people, their poor nutrition habits could be something that's been going on for years and years.

Thinking of things through that lens, it doesn't seem reasonable to go from 0 to 100 overnight. It also doesn't seem reasonable for things to go smoothly all of the time. Imagine someone who has suffered from addiction for years.

It's challenging for people to not slip up. This is why progress must be celebrated and you shouldn't harp on the slip-ups too much because it's likely that they will occur at some point.

Chapter 3: Executing Your Best Diet Game Plan

Now that you've been given a high-level overview of how you should be eating, I now want to give you some strategies for how we can put things in place to execute on this plan. I've talked about quite a few different things so far, and now is the time to put things together to help form a plan that can be executed.

Determining the Amount of Food that You Need to Eat

The first thing we need to figure out is the amount of food you need to eat to start improving your BMI. If you'll recall from earlier, you'll need to eat less calories than your metabolism burns off in order to lose weight. So how do you determine how many calories you burn off in a given day?

There are a lot of different formulas out there that you can use, but I like to keep things simple. Take your current body weight and multiply it by

13. This will tell you approximately how many calories you need to eat on a given day to sustain the weight you're currently at.

An example for someone who weighs 275 would be 275x13 for a total of 3,575 calories. Since the goal is to lose weight though, this person would need to eat less than 3,575 calories per day. The bigger the gap is between actual calories eaten and the maintenance number, the more weight that will be lost.

Meaning, if this person eats 2,575 calories per day, they will lose weight at a faster rate than if they eat 3,075 calories per day. There's no right or wrong approach to how quickly or slowly you should lose weight, but it is something you need to be thoughtful about. Losing weight faster may seem like the obvious choice, but there comes a point of diminishing returns.

You're going to be more miserable if you're eating less calories and it will make the plan harder to sustain. If you push the envelope too far, you'll push things over the edge, and your lymphedema symptoms won't see improvement. There's not going to be a way to know what pace is best for you until you experiment and find your groove.

I recommend starting smaller and working on eating less from there if you feel like you can handle it. Continuing with the example from earlier, if 3,575 calories would sustain that person's current weight, they could start off by eating 3,075 calories per day. This would equate to them losing about 1 pound per week.

If that seemed too challenging to maintain, they could bump the number up to 3,275 calories per day. If eating 3,075 wasn't too difficult, then they could push themselves a bit more and go for something like 2,875. Most people are ambitious in the beginning and that makes sense because we want change and we want it now.

The problem is you and your body have been used to eating a certain amount of calories per day for quite some time now. It's going to be a big adjustment to eat less than what your body is expecting to receive. In the beginning, you'll be fired up and likely won't have any issues.

As time goes on though, things will get tougher. Your motivation will fade, but the lower amount of calories will remain. This is why I believe it's better to start small and gradually decrease your calories.

This way the changes won't be noticed as heavily. So once you figure out your normal calories by taking your current body weight and multiplying it by 13, start by subtracting 250 from that number. Eat that many calories per day for a month and then eat a little bit less by subtracting 500 from your original number.

If you're a bit more ambitious, you could start off by subtracting 500, but remember we're playing the long game here. It does you no good to only do this for a month and then quit. You have to approach things in a way where you'll be able to do them theoretically for the rest of your life.

One Problem With This Approach

The thing I like about this method I just talked about is that it's simple to calculate. It's also good to measure data such as the calories you're eating because you'll know why you're making progress or why you're staying stuck. The problem can be with the execution.

I wouldn't exactly say that tracking the amount of calories in the foods you eat is fun. It wouldn't be a crazy stretch to say that most people don't like tracking their food intake, they'd just rather eat and not think about it. This is why I want to be realistic and give you a way you can go about things if you're not interested in tracking your calories.

Make no mistake about it though, it will be less accurate compared to someone who is willing to put in the extra effort to track things. So the choice is up to you. You could start by not tracking calories and seeing how that plays out with the advice I'm about to share.

If you don't make the kind of progress you want, you can then switch to tracking calories. Before I get into some advice on approaching things without tacking your calories, I first want to cover some ways to go about tracking your calories if that is something you're potentially interested in doing.

Using Technology to Track Your Calories

Luckily we live in a world where we can use technology to help us keep up with our calories. There are plenty of different apps that you can download to keep track of things. Most of them are the same with different interfaces, so I recommend trying out a few different ones and seeing what you like best.

My personal favorite is My Fitness Pal, but there are other good ones out there too. Regardless of what app you go with, you'll have a range of different options for how you want to track things. You can type in the food that you're eating and log it that way.

For instance, if you are eating half a cup of brown rice, you would type in brown rice, enter in the amount you are eating (which comes out to around 100 calories in this case), and log it as part of your meal. Boom, that's simple enough! Most calorie-counting apps also allow you to scan a barcode.

This will automatically pull up the nutritional information for that food, so you'll only need to focus on the amount that you ate. So how do you know how much of a certain food you ate? This is where you'll need to enlist the help of a food scale to help with your consistency.

It isn't hard to use a food scale as you can put your plate on the food scale and then zero it out. After that, you can put whatever the food item is on the plate and weigh the plate again. The difference is how many grams you'll be eating of that particular food.

It's not practical though to bring a food scale with you everywhere you go. So what do you do in cases where you're out and about and don't have access to your normal means of measuring such as a food scale? Well, one cool feature that some apps offer is the ability to take a picture of what you're eating and have the app tell you the calories.

This is usually a premium feature that you're going to have to pay for, but it will certainly make tracking easier. If you don't have access to this feature when you're out and about, then you'll simply need to take your best guess. If you're at a restaurant, then they'll sometimes have the nutritional information of their menu items online.

If you're at a party or something like that, you'll have to take an educated guess as to the amount of food that you're eating.

How to Go About Things if You Don't Want to Track Calories

Plenty of people who are in good health track their calories, but there are also plenty of other people in good health who never track their calories. So how can you go about things if you don't think tracking your calories is something that's sustainable for you? Well, something has to be tracked to ensure that you are making progress.

That measurement is going to be your weight. If you don't at the bare minimum step on the scale, then it's going to be hard to know if you're going in the right direction. Sure you could look at yourself in the mirror and see if you notice any changes.

The problem is that it takes a while for noticeable changes to be seen good or bad. That feedback won't occur frequently enough for it to be effective. You can easily measure your weight with a scale and it will tell us if what we're doing is working.

The trick is to measure your weight every day. Research shows that the simple act of measuring your weight every day can cause you to lose weight. This is because you're more aware of your weight and this will help you to make better food choices throughout the day.

It's the same premise of checking your bank account every day. You'll be more aware of your spending habits and thus make better choices simply because you're aware. The downside to weighing yourself every day is psychological.

Your weight will fluctuate on a daily basis meaning that you could weigh more tomorrow than you do today even if your eating is on point for the day. You have to be aware of this and take it for what it is. You need to view your weight from a zoomed-out perspective.

Over the weeks and months, has your weight gone down or up? If it's been 3 months and your weight hasn't changed, then that's reason for concern. If you weigh the same or even slightly more than you did yesterday, then you shouldn't stress about it.

You can use a simple spreadsheet to track your weight over time and it's something you should be doing regardless of if you're counting calories or not. Aside from tracking your weight, what should you do? Well, remember the advice I gave earlier about eating a certain percentage of your meals from healthy sources?

You want to follow this advice along with tracking your weight. So for instance, you might start off trying to eat 70% of your meals from clean sources and then improving your percentage week by week. If you eat 3 meals per day, this means you need to aim for about 15 of your meals to be wholesome.

You'll then track the number of healthy meals you're eating vs. unhealthy. You'll then compare this data against your weight. So let's say someone has a starting weight of 275 pounds with the goal of eating 15 of their 21 meals from healthy sources.

Let's say by the end of the week this individual ate 13 meals from clean sources and weighs 275.3. This means no weight was lost. The following week, the person would focus on improving his ratio such as from 13 meals to 15 and seeing if any weight loss occurs the following week.

Let's say the person ate 15 meals from healthy sources and still didn't lose any weight. The person could proceed from this point in one of two ways. The first option is to continue to improve on the healthy-to-unhealthy meal ratio and see if that improves things.

If the ratio continues to improve but weight loss remains stagnant, then you need to take a look at the volume of food you're eating during each of your meals. You want to focus your attention on cutting back slightly on some of your portion sizes and seeing if things improve. For example, when you eat an unhealthy meal, your portion size might be too large and this could be hindering your progress.

Looking to cut back on the portion sizes from your unhealthy meals will be the best place to start because calories from simple sugars and fats can add up quickly. So make simple changes where you can. Let's say you enjoy a fast food meal that consists of a cheeseburger, fries, and a soda.

You can improve on this meal by cutting out the cheese, getting a medium instead of a large, or skipping on the soda or fries. You don't have to fully optimize the meal to the point where you're not enjoying it, but you do want to aim to make at least one tweak. Make one small tweak such as cutting out the cheese from the meal.

Do one small change for each unhealthy meal that you eat and see if that tips the scale in the right direction. If it does, then great, continue doing what you're doing as long as weight loss continues. If weight loss still isn't occurring, then you're still eating too many calories.

Continue making small changes like I described until weight loss does occur. Yes, it can be frustrating to play the wait-and-see game, but it's the best you can do when you're not tracking your calories. Now let's say you get in a groove and you're losing weight, but then weight loss suddenly stops.

This is known as the dreaded weight loss plateau. It can be a tricky thing to navigate if you don't know what to do, so I want to ensure you're armed with the right knowledge to overcome it.

What to Do When Weight Loss Stalls

It's inevitable that as you start to lose weight, your progress will eventually slow down or stop altogether. It can be one of the most frustrating things to experience. Why can't things continue on the path that they have and you continue to lose weight?

When this happens, most people don't know how to handle it. This is where frustration will kick in and they'll be more likely to give up and gain all of their weight back that they worked so hard to lose in the first place. So why do weight loss plateaus occur in the first place?

Well, let's think about someone who weighs 275 pounds. Let's say this person loses 25 pounds and now weighs 250 pounds. The caloric needs of a 250-pound person are less than that of a 275-pound person.

There's more mass that needs to be maintained, which requires more energy, aka calories, to sustain. Therefore as you start to lose weight, you're changing your body's caloric needs. Remember the formula from earlier which was current bodyweight times 13 equals your maintenance calories.

For a 275-pound person, this comes out to 3,575. For a 250-pound person, this comes out to 3,250. So imagine if someone starts at 275 and starts eating less than 3,575 calories per day to start losing weight.

Specifically, let's say this person eats 3,250 calories per day. As they start losing weight, their caloric needs are decreasing and getting closer to the point where 3,250 is going to become their new caloric number to maintain their weight. Once that happens, weight loss will stop.

So when weight loss does stop, how do you overcome it? Well, you need to recalculate things because your caloric goals have changed. Let's say that person did go from 275 down to 250 but weight loss has screeched to a halt.
Now the person would need to use the formula again to recalculate their new caloric needs. In this case that would be 250 times 13 equals 3,250. That's the new maintenance number, which means the person needs to eat less than this.

Once the person starts eating less than this number, weight loss will resume again. This process needs to happen every time weight loss stalls, you essentially need to recalculate things. You don't need to obsess over this and recalculate every time you lose a pound or anything like that.

If things are working, then continue forward. Once things stop working, then you need to make an adjustment. Yes, this means that as you lose weight, you'll be eating fewer and fewer calories which isn't fun to think about.

However, I want you to stop and think about what your ideal weight is. If someone weighs 210 pounds and their goal is to weigh 150 to be at a healthy BMI, they simply don't need as many calories at that point. Plus this means that you're making progress, which is a good thing, so think of this in a positive way!

This is of course great and all if you're tracking your calories, but what if you're not tracking the amount of food that you're eating? Well, you'll still know if weight loss has stalled because you'll still be weighing yourself. Once you notice that your weight hasn't budged for a couple of weeks after you've seen good and consistent progress up to this point, then it's time to make a readjustment.

Start off by looking at your healthy-to-unhealthy meal ratio. See if there's room for improvement there. Maybe you're currently at 80% healthy meals, and you could try to take that up to 85%.

You could try to cut back in some way from meals that you're eating for enjoyment. So if you're eating at a restaurant, maybe you get water for your drink instead of a soda. You essentially want to follow more of the same advice I gave in the section about losing weight without tracking your calories.

Since you're not basing things off of numbers, the only way you'll know if you're making progress is to try out a change and see how it goes for you. The last piece of advice I want to give you when it comes to plateaus is to be patient with yourself. Overcoming a plateau isn't something that you can overcome in a day.

You have to make the necessary adjustments, see if they work, and then continue from there. Sometimes though your adjustments will not work, it will take some time to notice if the changes are working or not. If they aren't, then you have to continue to make adjustments, which takes time.

This is why it's important to be patient with yourself. If you've hit a plateau, consider it a good thing because this means that you've made progress from where you started to hit a plateau in the first place. When you get impatient, this is what will cause you to take drastic measures that will not be sustainable for the long haul. This is where you can create a bad cycle of gaining and losing weight all because you weren't willing to be patient with yourself and make methodical changes to the way that you're eating.

Chapter 4: Meal Prepping, Supplements, and Sample Meal Plan

By this point in the book, you have a good overall understanding of how you should eat and why you should eat in that way to best help out with lymphedema symptoms. However, there are still some things left unanswered that you might want to know. For one thing, you might want some sample meals to give you an idea of how you should be eating.

You also might be curious about supplements. Meal prepping might not be on your mind or maybe it is, but it's an essential step for success as you'll soon find out. By the end of this chapter, you should feel confident about taking the next steps forward to starting to lower your BMI. Let's kick things off by giving you an idea of how you should eat.

7-Day Sample Meal Plan

Monday

Meal 1: Oatmeal with Almond Milk and Honey, sides of Greek yogurt and blueberries

Meal 2: Spring Mix salad with olive oil dressing, salmon, and walnuts

Meal 3: Chicken breast with mashed potatoes and choice of green vegetable

Tuesday

Meal 1: Eggs and Turkey Bacon

Meal 2: Fruit smoothie consisting of blackberries, raspberries, blueberries, pineapple, and mango

Meal 3: Tacos using lean ground turkey and whole wheat tortillas with sides of brown rice and black beans

Wednesday

Meal 1: whole grain toast with natural peanut butter topped with raspberries and honey

Meal 2: Quinoa and Tuna with sides of green vegetables, pecans, and blueberries

Meal 3: Fajitas with whole wheat tortillas, green bell peppers, onions, and steak

Thursday

Meal 1: Protein shake with almond milk, Greek yogurt, oatmeal, blueberries, and plant-based whey protein

Meal 2: whole wheat pasta with lean ground beef, ground Turkey, or chicken

Meal 3: spring mix salad with lentils, raspberries, pecans, flax seeds and olive oil dressing

Friday

Meal 1: breakfast bowl consisting of eggs, ground Turkey, and hash browns

Meal 2: Protein Bowl consisting of chicken, brown rice, lentils, and guacamole

Meal 3: Enjoy a meal at a restaurant

Saturday

Meal 1: fruit smoothie consisting of whatever mix of fruit you want

Meal 2: Fast food meal of your choice

Meal 3: cauliflower crust pizza with turkey pepperoni

Sunday

Meal 1: breakfast from a doughnut shop or restaurant of your choice

Meal 2: roast beef stew with vegetables of your choice

Meal 3: pork chops with sweet potatoes and a green vegetable of your choice

So as you can see, 18 of the 21 meals are from healthy sources and would work towards helping you achieve your goals. The other 3 meals will allow you to have a nice break. In this example, I back-loaded the 3 meals towards the weekend, but your unhealthy meals can be dispersed however you choose.

18 out of 21 meals comes out to 85%, which is really good. Depending on where you're starting from, you may eat less than that percentage and that's completely okay. You'll just incorporate more meals from whatever you want throughout the week and work to improve from there.

Ultimately there's a lot of flexibility when it comes to the food choices you make. You don't always have to eat the same fruits and vegetables. There are plenty of different fruits and vegetables out there so you can switch it up regularly to avoid things getting stale.

The same thing goes for various types of nuts or protein sources that you may eat. You don't always have to eat chicken if you don't want to. You can switch things up accordingly based on what kind of protein sources that you do enjoy.

I wanted to provide a good amount of variety with this plan, but variety is by no means a necessity. You can stick with eating the same meals more frequently if you like eating the same things multiple times throughout the week.

Meal Prepping Your Way to Success

Eating healthy meals is great and of course most people want to eat healthier. So why doesn't it happen? Sure some foods can be bland and we would prefer to eat something else.

However, if there's a good healthy meal cooked and ready to eat most people won't mind. So why then don't people eat healthily more often even if their intentions are good? It comes down to being too busy and not being prepared.

You can have all of the motivation in the world and in the beginning, you will be highly motivated. You'll come home from work, ready to cook and prepare a healthy dinner. The problem is that as time goes on, your motivation will die down.

On top of that, you'll be coming home after a long day at work. You'll be tired mentally and physically. But now you don't have anything prepared for dinner.

In fact, you haven't even thought about what you want to eat. This is where people run into issues. You're now having to make a decision on what to eat when you're tired and hungry.

This is when poor decisions happen and you'll be more likely to get fast food. This way you won't have to think much about what to eat and you can have the meal prepared for you. This is something you'll be faced with time and time again.

Simply trying to fight against your fatigue is not a long-term winning strategy. You only have so much willpower to make decisions with throughout the day. In the morning your willpower will be at its highest.

As the day goes on and you have to make more and more decisions, your willpower will lessen. So when evening rolls around, you're behind the 8 ball if you don't know what you want to eat. This is why meal planning and prepping are so important for your success.

You can have the best diet plan out there but it doesn't matter if you're not able to follow through with it. So when it comes to meal prepping, there are different levels to it. The best-case scenario would be prepping as many of your meals ahead of time that you can.

I'll share my best tips for doing this, but you might not always be able to do this. This is why at the very least you want to know what you're eating ahead of time and make sure you already have all of the groceries you need to make the meal.

How Far in Advance Should You Plan Your Meals?

I believe it's best to plan out your meals one week at a time. This will help to ensure your prepped meals don't go bad and it will help to create a consistent routine for you. You can grocery shop on a weekly basis, and meal prep at certain times based on your work schedule.

You can pick any day that you want to prep your meals, but I've found some to work better than others. For me, I usually like to meal prep on Sundays. I don't have a lot going on and I mostly use this day for rest, relaxation, and getting ready for the upcoming week.

This gives me plenty of time to prep meals. Yes, it does take up a good chunk of time, but I'll usually have something on the TV or I'll listen to a podcast for entertainment while I prep. You could meal prep on a weekday, but I found this hard to do personally.

When you're tired, the last thing that's going to be on your mind is cooking for the rest of the evening. If there's a day that you're off and you have a good amount of free time, that's when you should try and prep. The very first step though is to plan out what meals you're going to eat.

So for every day of the week, for breakfast, lunch, and dinner, think about what you want to eat. Now the cool thing about planning is that you don't have to do this on the same day that you're going to prep. You could do it on Saturday and then shop and prep on Sunday for example.

Based on the meals you're going to eat, this will now determine what you need to buy at the grocery store. Once you have your groceries, I recommend batch-producing everything that you can. If you're eating 3 different meals that contain brown rice, then make 3 cups of brown rice.

If you're eating kale with every lunch as part of your side, then separate your kale across 5 containers so that it's ready to go for each day of the week. You'll notice that there are certain types of fruits or vegetables that you're going to be eating regularly throughout the week so you might as well prepare all of them ahead of time for the week. Also, consider foods that you can make at the same time.

If you have a rice cooker, you could start your rice. Then you could have a pot of boiling water to get ready to make some pasta while at the same time browning some lean beef. Thinking of ways in which you can knock out multiple food items in one swoop will really help to save time.

Some people like to split their meal planning up across two days such as a Sunday and a Wednesday. So you'd make as much food as you could for Monday, Tuesday, and Wednesday. Then on Wednesday evening, you'd make food for the rest of the week.

This never worked out that well for me because I found myself not having the time that I'd like to during the week to be able to meal prep. Life is unexpected and things can pop up during the evening that takes away your time from being able to prepare. You're suddenly left with going to bed late when you have to be up early for work or going to bed and being unprepared for the next day.

It's because of this unpredictability that I like prepping as much as I can for a week in advance. The last option that some people do is prepping their food on the previous day. So for example, you'd prepare Tuesday's meals on Monday and so on and so forth.

Again, I wouldn't consider this a consistent option because there's going to be too much variation during your evenings that will make it to where you might not be able to guarantee that you'll get around to prepping. Even if you do happen to have the time, there's no guarantee that you'll have the energy to prep for the next day. This is why I've found that prepping once a week is the best way to go about things.
Lastly, you want to think about containers. Containers are important because they can help to create consistency with your portion sizes. There are meal prep containers that are designed for a main dish and two sides.

So you could have your protein such as chicken as your main dish, and then green beans and mashed potatoes could be your two sides. Whenever you go to eat this meal again, you can create consistency with the amount of calories you eat because you'll only be eating as much as you're able to reasonably fit within the container.

This will ensure that you're eating a similar amount of mashed potatoes every time you eat that food for example. Then if you run into a situation where your weight loss has stalled, it will be easy to cut back on portion sizes if you have to because you could fill up that slot of your container with less mashed potatoes than you usually do.

Should You Take Any Supplements?

One common thing that people want to know about who want to improve their health is supplements. What supplements can someone take to help improve their overall health?

I totally understand the appeal as taking a supplement is easy to do, and if it benefits you, then why wouldn't you do it? In this case, when it comes to supplements, we need to look at supplements that can potentially help with lymphedema and supplements that can help with weight loss.

Supplements to Help with Lymphedema

Are there any supplements that can help you out with lymphedema? Well, there's not a ton of research out there to say that there's a supplement you should definitely be taking. And this brings me to my first point about supplements.

Everything I've discussed in this book up to this point is what will help you out the most. Therefore, that's what you should focus the majority of your attention on. You want to hone in on the things that will give you the biggest return and that's going to be what you eat and how much you eat in regards specifically to lymphedema symptoms and diet.

Think of supplements like the cherry on top. Sure it's a nice touch, but it's not the main part of the dessert. So don't expect any supplement to move mountains for you, but it doesn't hurt to try as long as you have the finances for a particular supplement.

If you don't, this isn't something to stress about because again you want to focus your attention on the meals you eat. You're going to eat multiple times a day every single day. If you're making poor decisions in that regard, there simply isn't going to be a pill that you can take once a day to help make up for that.

I want to help set the right expectations for this because people so often have the wrong mentality when it comes to this subject. If you approach things mentally with the understanding that nutrition is where your focus lies, then you'll be much better off. You'll come into things with proper expectations for what a particular supplement can and can not do for you.

So when it comes to lymphedema specifically, is there anything that should be on your radar? One thing that research has shown is that selenium levels tend to be deficient for individuals who have lymphedema and are obese. Selenium can help with inflammation, so it can be worth looking into to see if you're deficient in selenium and potentially supplementing with it.

What about weight loss supplements? Well, it's all about setting expectations once again. Don't expect anything that will be a magic bullet for you, but there are a few things you can look to for a small boost.

The first ingredient is something you could be taking already and that's caffeine. Research has shown that caffeine can boost your metabolism by a small amount. If your metabolism is faster, then you're burning more calories without having to do any additional work.

Regular intake could increase your metabolism by up to 8-11% over a period of time when caffeine is being taken, which is definitely something to think about. Another supplement to look into is carnitine. Carnitine has been shown to help increase weight loss by a small amount, so it can be worth taking for that boost.

Aside from these two supplements, is there anything else that could be recommended? Well, that's the thing there simply aren't a lot of good options out there when it comes to supplements that can legitimately aid in weight loss. Even the options I've listed so far give a small boost and that's it.

What's funny is there are plenty of commercials that lead you to think otherwise. You'll see these amazing before and after photos, and it will appear as if it's all because of this pill that they took. However, if you pay close attention you'll notice that they'll mention something about the pill being taken alongside a proper diet and exercise routine.

It may be in small print that you can't read, but you'll be able to find it if you look hard enough. And I think ironically enough that this sums up supplements perfectly. Even the people who are trying hard to sell you a weight loss supplement know that it can only do so much.

So don't buy into the hype of a particular weight loss supplement, stick to the basics of what I've mentioned here. There isn't a pill that can help you lose 30 or 50 pounds on its own. There are, however, things like caffeine and carnitine that can give you a small boost to help you out along the way so long as everything else you're doing is sound.

Now, there is one more supplement that I want to talk about, and it's not a weight loss supplement. However, in this case, since we're talking about lymphedema, one supplement that can be beneficial is fish oil.

Fish oil contains Omega-3 fatty acids which act as anti-inflammatories that we want to consume more of to help combat against the Omega-6 fatty acids that we consume. Essentially, you can help ensure that you're consuming enough Omega-3 fatty acids in your diet by taking a fish oil pill or consuming the liquid.

Finally, as we are drawing near to the end of this book, would you mind taking a little bit of time and leaving a review? It would mean a lot to me and I will value your feedback.

Conclusion

Dealing with lymphedema is not a fun thing. It's even more unfortunate that there isn't a cure for it, but that doesn't mean that there aren't things you can do to help make the most of the situation. There are exercise and massage routines that you can follow, but diet is not something that should be overlooked.

The old phrase really is true, you are what you eat. We eat every day and it's not something that we can avoid. This is why it's so important to be able to make the proper choices regarding nutrition on a day-to-day basis but do so in a way that doesn't feel like pure drudgery all of the time.

This is why I believe implementing meals that you know you'll enjoy is a very important step for your success. If you're able to properly strike this balance in a way that works for you, you'll be able to sustain this for a long time to come, and that's the real key to seeing and sustaining success when it comes to your diet.

References

https://www.ncbi.nlm.nih.gov/pmc/articles/PMC6237444/

https://www.ncbi.nlm.nih.gov/pmc/articles/PMC2965625/

https://pubmed.ncbi.nlm.nih.gov/33493081/#:~:text=As%20BMI%20increases%20lymphedema%20worsens,to%20reduce%20complications%20and%20recurrence.

https://pubmed.ncbi.nlm.nih.gov/25683820/#:~:text=Conclusions%3A%20Weighing%20every%20day%20led,an%20effective%20weight%20loss%20tool.

https://pubmed.ncbi.nlm.nih.gov/32359762/#:~:text=Conclusions:%20l%2Dcarnitine%20supplementation%20provides%20a,body%20weight%2C%20BMI%20and%20fat

https://pubmed.ncbi.nlm.nih.gov/2912010/#:~:text=Single%2Ddose%20oral%20administration

%20of,observed%20in%20the%20postobese%2
0subjects.

https://www.ncbi.nlm.nih.gov/pmc/articles/PM
C7281982/

https://www.ncbi.nlm.nih.gov/pmc/articles/PM
C5297803/#:~:text=Lymphedema%20results%2
0from%20lymphatic%20insufficiency,overall%2
0poor%20quality%20of%20life.